POWER WOMAN

JOY ONYESOH

Original Cover Design: Kadesh Ministry Design And Media

Intern: Jerome Totten

Special thanks to our editing teams

Printed in the United States of America

Foreword

Joy is as an activist, a fierce defender of women's rights, a feminist sister, and a compassionate filled woman. Over the years of knowing Joy, I have come to know a person who is gentle, yet fierce; a person who is kind yet uncompromising. As an African woman, Joy understands the complexity of the African culture as relates to women's empowerment. Even with the persistence of said complexities, Joy is marvelously determined to change the narrative for women's empowerment within her community and the world. As a friend and sister of Joy, I marvel at her ability to salvage the stories of women from different parts of the world and turn them into a cornerstone for women's growth.

Let's face the fact- not many books are written solely for women, our experiences, and our development. More to this is the uncanny truth that when stories about women's well-being are told, they are told from a man's perspective. Joy's narration of personal and shared women's stories in Power Woman, especially African women is inexplicably rare. It unprecedentedly provides a guide for women on ways to navigate their personal journey. Growing up as an African woman, we did not have many books like Power Woman, but Joy has changed that narrative for our young daughters and women . No longer will they have to search for themselves in places they are not welcomed and celebrated.

In Joy's words, women will learn about the journey of other strong women. They will read the stories of adaptability, forgiveness, emotion, betrayal, focus and advancement. In Power Woman, women, from all walks of life, will gain a new understanding of strength as in this book, Joy teaches us women to be strong, but not strong in the way the world tells us. Joy's portrayal of strength is powerful, relatable- she shows us lived examples in personal journey. Through her personal experiences and path to forgiveness, to divine grace, Joy explores a new meaning of faith. Faith in a way that empowers all women, regardless of race, status and creed to take on the world and achieve their goal. Joy's words enact a new meaning of consciousness.

I am excited to watch Power Woman transform the lives of many individuals. I am excited to see women irrespective of their age begin their life's journey with Power Woman.

ABOUT LEYMAH GBOWEE

Foreword Writer for Power Woman

2011 Nobel Peace Laureate Leymah Gbowee is a Liberian peace activist, trained social worker and women's rights advocate.

She is the founder and current President of the Gbowee Peace Foundation Africa. Her foundation provides educational and leadership opportunities to girls, women and youth in West Africa in order to raise the next generation of peacebuilders and democratic leaders. She currently serves as Executive Director of the Women, Peace and Security Program at Columbia University's Earth Institute. Ms. Gbowee was the founding head of the Liberia Reconciliation Initiative, and co-founder and former Executive Director of Women Peace and Security Network Africa (WIPSEN-A). She was also a founding member and former Liberian Coordinator of Women in Peacebuilding Network/West Africa Network for Peacebuilding (WIP-NET/WANEP). She travels internationally to advocate for human rights and peace & security.

Ms. Gbowee's leadership of the Women of Liberia Mass Action for Peace – which brought together Christian and Muslim women in a nonviolent movement that played a pivotal role in ending Liberia's civil war in 2003 – is chronicled in her memoir, *Mighty Be Our Powers*, and in the award-winning documentary, *Pray the Devil Back to Hell*. She holds an M.A. in Conflict Transformation and many honorary doctorate degrees.

Ms. Gbowee is an advisor for numerous organizations. She serves as a member of the UN Secretary General's High-Level Advisory Board on Mediation, the World Refugee Council and the African Women's Leadership Network. Ms. Gbowee is a member of the prize committees of two major humanitarian awards: the Aurora Prize for Awakening Humanity and the Conrad N. Hilton Humanitarian Prize. In 2020, Ms. Gbowee joined the Higher Committee of Human Fraternity, a multi-faith committee dedicated to fostering peaceful coexistence through dialogue. Ms. Gbowee was a member of the G7 Gender Equality Advisory Council during Canada's G7 Presidency in 2018 and is an alumni of the UN's Sustainable Development Goals Advocates.

Ms. Gbowee has been named as one of the Top 100 Most Influential People in Gender Policy by Apolitical and one of the World's 50 Greatest Leaders by Fortune Magazine.

***

Prologue

During the writing of my first book, *The Moulding of the Master's Vessel: Our Journey With Brittle Bone Disease*, I encountered deep emotions and had to pause during the writing process. Some emotions I had to deal with were that of anger and pain. I realized that I had not forgiven certain persons for their actions and their words spoken to me while nurturing my daughter, who is living with brittle bone disease. I had uncovered a wound so deep that I needed to deliberately ensure that I had stopped bleeding inside. I had to let the pain go. Thus, I took a series of positive actions towards helping me heal my wounds. I then returned to writing and finishing my book. I made a commitment to write another book that will focus on forgiveness, self-discovery, emotions and personal growth.

This is that book.

This book is inspired by my experience nurturing and caring for my daughter living with a rare medical condition called Brittle Bone. I had to navigate the deep oceans of pain, guilt, a sense of betrayal by family and friends but found peace in the transformative power of forgiveness. I learnt to forgive others and myself and I share life lessons of my transformative journey in this book. This is my second book following, *The Moulding Of the Master's Vessel.* This book is aimed at facilitating a deep understanding of forgiveness, how to deal with pain and inner wounds and the importance of living a healthy and limitless life.

I share the gift of healing and growth that forgiveness brought into my life and I pray for those hurting because they can't bring themselves to forgive themselves or others. I pray that they will come to a point of realization that the past can only hold you down if you are not willing to let go and embrace the freedom of a future filled with possibilities.

I delve into my transformative personal growth, sharing some life experiences that will motivate and inspire you to be the best version of yourself.

CONTENTS

1

Understanding Forgiveness

Forgiveness means different things to different people. However, it involves a decision to let go of resentment and is an art that requires a deep consciousness and heightened level of self-awareness, the grace of God, deep-rooted positive relationship with the self and love. I write about forgiveness from a place of commitment to a personalized process of growth, grace and deep commitment to continuously shed the weight and burden. It is difficult to heal when the emotions about an incident or process are so strong and no conscious effort is made to understand the depth and moving beyond the betrayals or pain.

My daughter was diagnosed with a rare congenital disease called brittle bone also known as Osteogenesis Imperfecta

(OI), this is a condition that is characterized by frequent fracture of the bones especially the long bones and the severity varies from mild to very severe depending on the type of OI the child has. It can be a very traumatic process for parents, family members, and the child. When I was confronted with this information, I felt that life was meaningless and held no hope for my child and I, and this made me so scared. In my fear, I didn't consider the fact that I had two healthy kids and that the future could hold hope. Instead, I focused on the fact that the disease has no cure and I blamed myself for her condition. These feelings manifested into internal wounds. My self - torturing worsened every single minute of the day.

One of my regular reactions was to focus on caring for my daughter to the detriment of my own health. I felt that I had to pay the penance for allowing her to have this condition. Each time she had a fracture the cycle of guilt, resentment, and unforgiveness would rear its ugly head.

The second manifestations that I had was that of shying away from engaging in anything constructive as I had developed low self-esteem from the feelings of failure. I couldn't forgive myself, I couldn't allow my life to go on smoothly while my daughter was lying in pain. I understand clearly now that life comes in various shades for each one of us. There are certain challenges that no matter how much you prepare for them, you can never understand the dimension of the pain, guilt, loss, or any other emotion that come with it until you experience it. You'll never know your exact reaction until you are in it.

The key thing to understand here is that forgiveness is a process and there are situations that will require you to practice the art of either interpersonal or intrapersonal forgiveness. I had to start with myself first; which is interpersonal forgiveness.

Identify Your Hurt

One way of moving forward in your forgiveness journey is by pinpointing the source of your hurt. It is important to acknowledge your hurtful emotions. What is your pain about? Is it a failure, a missed opportunity, a heartbreak, loss of a loved one, ill health, a person who was mean to you, or someone who neglected you? Get to the root of your pain. Know exactly how you feel about what happened and be able to articulate what you are feeling. Is it sadness, grief, anger, pity, or loneliness? Or is it something deeper like hate, disgust, jealousy, or depression? The hurt may strike more than one chord on your heartstrings, but to get rid of the hurt, you need to recognize your feelings toward it.

I've realized that forgiveness is a process and requires patience and commitment. We define a process as: a series of actions or steps required to achieve a particular end, and in this case, the end is forgiveness. This means that forgiveness requires a level of awareness to facilitate the transformation required. This involves being patient with yourself, understanding that the hurt or grudge that made you feel resentful would need to be acknowledged and dealt with positively.

Get the Right Perspective on What is Happening

I can vividly recall how resentful and sensitive I was after my daughter's medical diagnosis. The thought of me being primarily responsible for her condition made me feel so resentful towards myself. It was a process of self-discovery, patience, and reaching out that kick-started my forgiveness process. Some pains are more deeply rooted than others and to heal and have the freedom to move forward you need to **give yourself the permission to heal.**

I remember one of the young girls that I counseled, who at a young age experienced the pain of watching both parents consistently quarrel with each other. The moments of expressed love were few and far between; often accompanied by another lengthy period of quarreling and fighting. The young lady said that her young mind didn't understand why both parents couldn't just laugh together and be as happy as her friends' families. In time both parents' misunderstandings got so complicated and they had to get a divorce. The young lady said she was outwardly very calm but inwardly shaken. She felt ashamed to discuss what she was experiencing with anyone or to mention the fact that her parents were divorced. She felt that perhaps she could have prevented both parents from separating. She didn't realize how deeply rooted her sense of guilt was until she started dating. She didn't want her relationship to end up like that of her parents and felt that if she tried hard enough, if she could endure more, maybe her partner would try hard as well. This led to a lot of expectations and of course, she couldn't keep a healthy relationship and went from one unhealthy relationship to the other. She was badly hurt and developed a sense of low self-esteem and low confidence. She had built up a lot of anger and resentment and she became depressed. She was very upset with God and had stopped attending church because she felt that there was no need for fellowship. She was invited for a singles program, which she reluctantly attended but later said that she felt the program was designed specifically for her. That was how she started her healing journey. She learned to forgive herself, let go, and began a new journey of freedom.

Often **forgiveness is required internally** before it becomes manifest externally; I say this from a place of experience. I had to learn how to forgive myself and then extend that to others who hurt or betrayed me consciously or unconsciously. By choosing to forgive and letting go, you release yourself from the power these individuals or situations hold over you, build healthier relationships, have improved self-esteem, less anxiety, less stress and improved mental health. Compassion and empathy materialize into action when you forget about the problem and move on to the space of forgiveness. Give your forgiveness to that person, with no strings attached. **It is your gift to yourself.** Instead of mentally replaying your hurt, seek fresh ways to get what you want. Remember that a life well-lived is your best revenge. Instead of focusing on your wounded feelings, and thereby giving the person or situation power over you, learn to look for the love, beauty, and kindness around you. Forgiveness is about personal power and agency. Remind yourself that you have the power to achieve and get all that you need.

2

Understanding and Balancing Emotions

Forgiveness involves feelings and attitudes. Our feelings warn us when things go wrong and they are God-given. When we feel hurt by the actions of someone, in itself it is not wrong or a bad thing, but it is what we do with the feelings and how we manage the feelings that make the difference. We need to know that the emotions won't just go away and we must also not deny the feelings or feel guilty about them, rather we must determine to deal with it positively.

Understanding

To deal with our emotions, we must prepare to be in it for the long haul. The first part of dealing with your emotions is understanding them. Understanding your emotions has to do with comprehension, mastery, and having insight. There is a need to interrogate your emotions, to have a comprehensive idea of the actions or situations that are making you feel bitter or that elicits negative emotions from you. The process of comprehension may be difficult and slow but commit to the untangling that needs to happen. It is difficult to move forward without having a good insight as to what you need to declutter and let go of. When you are hurt, at times you may feel vengeful and would want similar pain or even pain worse that what you are feeling to be felt by the erring party. Deep-rooted pain, which stems from the action or inaction of others, can be very difficult to deal with without help and guidance. Proverbs 3:5-6 (NIV) states, **"Trust in the Lord with all your heart and lean not on your own understanding; in all your ways submit to him, and he will make your paths straight."**

Trusting in the Lord brings a deeper insight into the situation and gives you a good foundation to interrogate your emotions.

I remember in the early days of nurturing my daughter, I was constantly feeling angry with everyone. I even felt so bitter with God. For I couldn't understand how he could watch my daughter go through indescribable pains. These intense bitter emotions made me experience intense mood swings. I was moving from one extreme emotion to the other effortlessly. I recognized that the emotions and mood swings were not helping me; rather it was draining my energy. I knew that if I wanted to feel better (because I was tired of feeling hurt, angry and bitter), I would need to make a deliberate effort to seek help. The first place I went to was to cry unto God. One of those times my daughter had one of her fracture episodes, I broke down in complete surrender, asking God for the grace to keep moving on. I couldn't see any future in our current circumstances. I was blaming everyone around me, including myself. It was not a pleasant place to be in. It was one of my very dark moments. The book of Prov 3: 5-6 became a comforting passage to me. Each time I felt myself sinking into those mood swings, I cried out to God for help. I was never tired of seeking His face or drawing towards His grace. Dwelling in His presence became my comfort. The healing I drew from those encounters strengthened my trust and faith. Sometimes, when I had doubting moments, I wondered if God was seeing my pains and why He couldn't just heal my emotions. I was just so tired of the emotional rollercoaster. I had deep inner wounds, which came from a lot of spaces and incidents. Nurturing my daughter brought to the forefront of the emotional issues that I had yet to deal with. But I had to start dealing with all those emotions, I had no other option and I could no longer deny that I needed help. It takes a lot of courage to open up yourself to dealing with your emotions.

It requires tenacity and resilience to move beyond the pain and to start the journey of healing. The journey of healing doesn't always feel good, but the results make it all worth it.

Forgiveness is a Choice

Forgiveness should come from a place of love, hope, and strength. The first place is to start by forgiving yourself. You may ask why do I need to forgive myself? I recently lost my older brother and it is one of my most painful experiences. I am still on the journey of healing and recovery, however each day that passes brings me to a more comforting space. His death was a shock that threw me off, challenged my faith and caused an outpouring of emotions that I never thought possible. I was oscillating between numbness, pain and desperately trying to hold on to my faith and trust in God. He transitioned to glory while I was away on an official business trip. I had a series of back-to-back travels that lasted for close to three weeks. As usual, I had called him and then went over to spend some time with him before I left, as I knew that I would be away for a while. We agreed we would see each other upon my return. Little did I know that would be to be my last physical encounter with him. While I was away, he took ill and a lot of complications followed the process which led to his death. The night he passed on I had a dream that got me so worried and I called home. Even though I was told that he was much better but was sleeping, I felt so uneasy. I lost my peace from that day until I came back into the country. Upon my return, I was confronted with the painful news and reality of his death. My pain and grief knew no bounds. Then the guilty feelings settled in, I wished I hadn't traveled; I felt if I had been around that I would have managed the situation better. All the things that I could have done if I had been there came tumbling in and I felt that I had let him down.

Even when my immediate family members and close friends were telling me, I did all that was humanly possible, it still didn't hold waters for me. I felt that I should have been on the ground. The fact is even if I were on the ground it wouldn't have changed anything. He fought a good fight, and it was his time to go. We did all that we could, and he was surrounded by love till the end.

You may have endured a similar situation. Battling with the loss of a loved one is never easy. The wounds may still be raw and bleeding. You've refused to forgive yourself for being absent or not taking quick action or some other thoughts that you could have prevented the death or done something differently while your loved one was alive. Listen, you need to give yourself the permission to forgive yourself and move on. You made the best decision that you could at that point in time and if you felt that you still could have done more it's all in the past and you can't re-write the past. However, you can be more intentional and deliberate in the future. Don't allow the pain or guilt to hold you down that you lose yourself in the process. Forgiveness is a choice; it's your gift to yourself. Draw from it and be kind to yourself.

I had to learn how to trust the Lord with my entire heart and not to lean on my own understanding. This was really an untangling process. I had to take one step at a time completely believing in God to help me in resolving my emotions. I was also committed to the process and willing to see it through.

One challenge we have in understanding our emotions is that we expect the process to be quick and easy. We want instant results and emotional healing and we get frustrated when we don't get the expected results. It is helpful to remember that no matter what, no matter how long it takes, you can't give up. You must remain too focused to give up. I coined my mantra; **"Too Focused To Give Up"** when I was deep in one of my many struggles. It has helped me overcome and persevere during the hard times and I hope it does the same for you too.

I Forgive You But ...

Some people like to take advantage of others, especially when you are perceived as a believer, a kind-hearted or understanding person. Deliberate premeditated hurtful actions will be carried out on you and or hurtful emotional words will be thrown at you and there is the expectation that you should forgive and forget and carry on as if nothing happened. In some cases, you won't be granted the freedom to express how you feel. This may be because of the consequences or that the space is not healthy or safe for such expression.

More frequently we are witnessing a rise in intimate partner crime, violence against women and girls and other forms of gender-based violence. We live in a society where patriarchy reigns supreme and impunity is the order of the day. Babies, girls, women are violated with impunity, our young boys are not left out either. News of recurrent and consistent domestic violence pervades all levels. Some women are afraid to speak up because of the culture of silence around violence against women and girls. In conflict communities, women and girls become soft targets for both the state military and the militants. Survivors are often asked to forgive the perpetrator and move on. The idea of forgiveness that is requested from the survivors is to let the perpetrator go off without any punitive actions taken. I want to remind us that our God is one of justice and if violators are allowed to roam free, then so many more women and girls would be in danger. Forgiveness does not imply that when one commits a criminal offense such a person is to be aided to evade the punitive measures prescribed by law.

Lean Not on Your Own Understanding

The pain of being hurt or disappointed could build up into a feeling of fear. You become scared of living because you think something bad will happen or you get overprotective of a loved one because of your painful experience. **Fears are normal human emotions created by our imagination to make reality seem scarier than it is.** Learning to deal with fear is all about putting your negative thoughts in perspective. We focus too much on the negative, so by looking at all the options, you often realize that you're making an enormous deal out of nothing. There are so many things that can happen that it's impossible for you to predict them all, so why even try? Getting through fear is a skill that you can learn. If you aren't ready to face your fears, you probably won't transcend them. Before you can begin managing your fear, you must understand that **you are not your fears. You are the awareness that experiences it.** The Bible provides wonderful support for one going through fear and finding ways of breaking free. Going back to the book of Proverbs, it reminds us to **"Trust in the Lord with all your heart and lean not on your own understanding..."** (Proverbs 3:5 NIV)

What does it mean to lean not on your own understanding? Most of us have a desperate desire to understand, but in so many areas we must acknowledge that we cannot understand. We often will not understand *how* God is causing **"all things to work together for good"** (Romans 8:28 NIV) But when we trust Him with all our hearts, we know that He *is God* and He will never fail us. Trusting in the Lord to heal your emotions and acknowledging that He alone can direct your path is a positive step forward in creating an enabling environment for inner peace and healing to occur.

3

Feeling Stuck

"It's All Perception! When we feel stuck, going nowhere even starting to slip backward — we may actually be backing up to get a running start."

- Dan Millman

There are periods in life when you feel like you've tried everything to improve your life, but nothing changes. The feeling of frustration sets in because you feel that everything seems to work against you and before long your confidence dips. Allow me to put your mind at ease. Feeling stuck is only a perception and does not represent your actual reality. It does, however, signal that something needs to change in your life. You might have an intuitive impulse to make those changes, but resist doing so for fear of change and perhaps your feeling of not being enough to create the change you want to see.

I remember some years back; I felt that I was stuck at a point and I wasn't growing the way I desired. I had this earnest desire to help women discover their purpose and to live a life of limitless possibilities. However, every plan I made to get me started off was in the wrong direction, or so it seemed. I got to a point of frustration as I felt I was investing a lot of energy and time. At some point confusion set in, as I couldn't actually pinpoint the right path to follow. I knew deep inside of me that my life experiences and professional qualification positioned me to be of service to women who were going through life struggles, self -doubt, and low self-esteem. One day during my morning devotion, while reading Job 22:28 NIV **"Thou shalt also decree a thing, and it shall be established unto thee; and light shall shine upon thy ways."** The words literally jumped at me. I felt this surge of excitement knowing that the first thing I need to do is to decree what I want. I needed to make a pronouncement. It was important that I had a vivid vision of what I wanted for my life and how I can be of service to humanity, which was my earnest desire. I instantly knew that if I could do this, it meant that my Father would establish it and I only have to trust Him to do what He has promised. That was an enormous mindset shift. I started perceiving my challenges with a new mindset. I knew that I had to stop trying too hard, so much so that I boxed myself into a corner. I realized that the harder I tried the less I am likely to see results, due to a change in conditions that have now progressed. It was important that I step back and view my situation or challenges from a wider perspective, armed with the infallible promises of God to establish all that I shall decree. The difference now is that I struggle less, because I'm beginning to let go and allow God to lead me to the right path. I finally realized that it's how I perceive the situation that makes me "feel stuck".

What is that situation or challenge that is making you feel overwhelmed and stuck? Perhaps it's time to relax and surrender and understand that you can't control life but you can control your reaction to what life brings to you.

I have learnt to do the best I can with what I have. I must say that it's not easy being a mother of a special needs child, especially when the condition is a very rare disorder. There was a time it made me so mad that we had to go through the pain and uncertainty but I look at where we are right now and I am filled with so much gratitude. I've learnt to make the most of the moments. It is in the darkest periods of my life that I discovered the most about myself and built my resilience.

I've learned that life isn't all about accomplishing things sometimes it's about resting and letting things be. Life happens in seasons. We all experience change and transition in life. Sometimes life is exciting, dynamic, and we feel on top of the world. At other times we just want to go away and escape the situation. So it's important that we understand the seasons so we do not draw the wrong conclusions about what is happening in our lives, or the reasons for it.

How to overcome feeling stuck

At times we feel stuck because we are trying to hang onto something that is in the past. My advice is don't try to push something in the wrong season, quit looking back all the time wishing for your favorite season of the past to return. Instead we must forget what lies behind and push forward to what lies ahead. The future is filled with limitless opportunities and we must learn to embrace it . Be consistent and do the work that the season you are in requires and learn from every season that you are in. Every season has lessons of life for us. Remember that we can't control what happens around us, but we can control what happens inside. You can't control how people treat you, but you can control how you respond to what they do.

Positive Steps to push you forward.

In this section, I have added some space for you to write in your personal responses. This will help you gain deeper clarity and purpose.

- Things change because your perception changes. Be kind to yourself and give yourself permission to take one baby step at a time.
  I, _____, give myself permission to take one baby step at a time.

- Let go and enjoy yourself. There's always something you feel drawn to do during these periods. You're not completely stuck, not in every area of your life. Do the work you need to do. But then give yourself the permission to have fun.

Things I can do for fun are...

1.

2.

- Quit being anxious. You cannot control everything, so you need to learn to just let go of some things. Learn to relax and take things easy. You may be feeling stuck because you are always in your own head obsessing and worrying.

Today I will stop worrying about ...

1.

2.

- Spend time with yourself discovering you. Invest in your self-awareness and don't allow whatever situations you are going through define you. You need to set boundaries and teach people how to value you and your choices.

Today I will take baby steps to set boundaries regarding...

1.

2.

- Writing gives me clarity and helps ease my tension. At times when I feel truly stuck, I write. I journal everything going on in my head. No holds barred, no censoring. I just keep writing. I formed this habit at a very early age. I learnt to put into words my feelings and thoughts. It's very therapeutic for me and I am encouraging you to form that habit of writing whenever you feel stuck. It may help you declutter your thoughts and untangle all the complex feelings. The more aware you become, the more these things fall away. When you truly become aware of what goes on inside of your head, you start to let go and learn to focus on more positive things. Remember energy grows where energy flows. If you build the habit of intentionally being positive about challenging times, you will experience a mindset shift.

Can you commit to journaling at least once a week? Why or why not? And if not journaling, what else can you do to help clear your mind and get your thoughts out weekly?

_____

_____

_____

_____

_____

_____

- You may think that there is nothing substantial you can do to change your situation. Even the tiniest possible step is progress. Focus on baby steps, enjoy and celebrate your micro wins. This gives you the confidence to look up and stand tall to tackle bigger issues. If you are reading this and you are feeling stuck, I encourage you to start right now, make a list of tiny ways you can get closer to your goal of feeling unstuck. Then pick one and act on it as soon as possible. The thing with feeling stuck is that sometimes you don't know what you need to get unstuck. You don't need to have it all figured out to move forward. I tell you this from experience, just remain committed to taking one baby step at a time. Clarity will come from you taking consistent positive action. Even if you cannot envision the end result and don't know where it is exactly that you're going, it is crucial to just start moving. Keep taking small actions until you figure out what it is that you want and how to get it.

What are some small actions you can take?

_____

_____

_____

_____

_____

- You need to believe in yourself. You are more than enough to ride out whatever situation that you are going through and believe in what your heart tells you, not what others say. Remember that it's YOUR life. You need to be on the driver's seat and intentionally navigate your journey.

Write out 5 positive things you love about yourself...

1.

2.

3.

4.

5.

SECTION II

4

P.O.W.E.R
WOMAN

For you to intentionally navigate your journey, you need to be a P.O.W.E.R woman that is focused and ready to evolve into your purpose. It doesn't matter what you've been through, it doesn't matter how battered and downcast you are. What matters is your commitment to yourself and you giving yourself the permission to play full out. No one says it would be an easy process but the truth is if you don't believe in yourself and value your dream so deeply that you lose your sleep until you birth it, no one else will do that for you. You set the pace in teaching others how to value you and how best to support you.

Some years back I came across T.D Jakes book "*Woman Thou Art Loosed*". By the way, I love the way T.D Jakes is so invested in giving women visibility and supporting women to own their truth and their journey. Through his book, I learnt valuable lessons on knowing and owning my uniqueness. Perhaps you are at a point in your life when you are questioning the essence of your life and wondering if life could be any worse. I am here to remind you that you have the key to your freedom. It is time to take stock and take control of your life. Are you ready to step out? This reminds me of the song "I am coming out" By Diana Ross. This song topped the charts and is the most successful solo by Diana Ross. Do you wonder why? It is a highly motivational song that moves one to break barriers and be the best version of oneself. In the song Diana talks of coming out and wanting the world to know her, to experience her as a gift and she really did. In that song she spoke about the power of positivity, the need to give back to the world, to show her abilities. She also spoke of spreading love and not fear. This song typifies a P.O.W.E.R Woman.

I will share five secrets for coming out, being the best version of yourself and living a life of abundance. These secrets are encapsulated in the acronym P.O.W.E.R

- Principled

- Organized

- Wealthy

- Empathetic

- Resilient

Secret # 1: Principled

What really are principles and how does it transform your life? Why should a POWER Woman be principled? Too often we hear people say oh Mrs. XYZ is principled. Under this subhead we would dig deeper into unraveling principles and developing a personal set of principles to guide you through your life journey.

Principle is a concept or proposition that serves as the foundation for a system of belief or for a chain of reasoning. Developing your principles is one of the core activities that you need to invest in if you want to live a life of abundance and of e limitless possibilities.

Your principles are like your compass. They guide you in the direction that you should travel. Can you stop for one minute and imagine what would happen if you have no compass directing your journey? No prepared traveler goes on a journey in an uncharted course without having clear directions. If you have the wrong map for your life travels you will end up in unintended places and these can have dire consequences.

For some people some of the challenges they currently face can be traced to not having a clear direction as to where they intend to end up.

STEPS IN DEVELOPING PRINCIPLES

Articulate Your Values

Values are what guides or motivates your actions and attitudes. They determine what is important to you and provide a general guideline for your conduct.

According to R.K. Mukherjee[1], "Values are socially approved desires and goals that are internalized through the process of conditioning, learning or socialization and that become subjective preferences, standards, and aspirations". While I. J. Lehner and N.J. Kube[2] and, "Values are an integral part of the personal philosophy of life by which we generally mean the system of values by which we live. The philosophy of life includes our aims, ideals, and manner of thinking and the principles by which we guide our behavior".

I appreciate the two definitions of values given above and one can summarily say that the values are:

1. Socially constructed

2. Internalized through our socialization process

3. Subjective

---

[1] R.K. Mukherjee (1951). Values and Value Orientations in the Theory of Action' In T. Parsons & E.A. Shils (Eds),'Toward A General Theory of Action' Harvard University Press, Cambridge.

[2] http://ijics.com/gallery/8-mar-929.pdf INCULCATION OF VALUE EDUCATION IN TEACHER EDUCATION

4. Integral to principles

5. Guides our actions and thought process

6. Contains interpretations of right or wrong

7. Guides our perception

From the above you can understand the importance of having the right set of value systems. It determines how far you can soar in life.

Sources of Values are:

- **Family:** This is the first socialization unit a child is introduced to and the family is a great source of values. A child learns his first value from his family.

- **Friends & Peers:** An impactful source of values is from peers and friends. This is why you must be intentional as to who you surround yourself with. You can pick up values unconsciously by being in the wrong cycle just as you can also pick up positive values. Choose your circle of friends intentionally.

- **Community:** As a part of community, a person learns values from community or different groups of within the community

- **Educational Institutions:** Educational institutions also play a very important role in introducing values.

- **Media:** Media such as – Print media, Social media, Electronic media also play the role of increasing values in the mind of people. They are used for re-orientation and shaping perceptions. These days for some job interviews and visa application interviews, you are asked to share your social media handles. This helps in peeking into your life and the shared values that you have.

- **Religion:** To a large extent religion shapes your perception and guides your actions or attitudes. Religious leaders are seen as influencers because the role they play in values internalization is recognized.

- **Books:** Engaging with the right set of books can shape your value system.

Of course the list above is not an exhaustive one, there are many other sources for values. Use this as a foundation to help be more understanding of how your environment impacts you.

How to Identify Your Values

Oftentimes, when I give a talk on values and the importance of our values I get questions on how to identify personal values. You can use the extra space on this page or get your own piece of paper to do the following exercise. The exercise below will get you started and keep you on course in identifying your core values.

- Brainstorm all the characteristics; feelings, behaviors or qualities that you know of examples include integrity, honesty, transformative leadership etc.

- Prune the list down to ten. Eliminate words that are encapsulated by others or have shared meanings.

- Describe the values and what they mean to you.

- Arrange the values in order of priority and select the core 5 values that are uniquely you.

_____

_____

_____

_____

_____

_____

Congratulations! You have identified your core values and are ready for the next step in developing your principles.

The second step in developing your principles is to identify your personal value proposition.

What is your Personal Value Proposition (PVP)? It is the foundation for living a limitless life of possibilities. It is everything in a job search, career progression and personal development. It helps in attracting the help of others, and explaining why you're the one to pick, the one to hire and not someone else. It speaks to who you are and what you represent.

Four Steps to Developing a PVP

1. Set a Clear Target. Targeting makes you most effective. You can't serve everyone and you can't be all things. Your Personal Value Proposition begins with a target, one that needs what you have to offer. Who do you serve primarily? I serve passionate women who are willing to give themselves permission to play full out and are willing to invest in themselves so as to live a life of limitless possibilities. This doesn't mean that I don't serve other audiences. However, this is my primary target and I develop myself to be positioned to serve the needs of this set of women. This gives me fulfillment.

2. Identify your strengths. It may sound obvious, but what you know and what you can do is the foundation of your PVP. Identify, concentrate, and hone in on what those are.

3. Tie your strengths to your target position. It is up to you to sell yourself once you figure out what your strengths are. How does your strength relate to what your target needs? If you are in business, you need to tie in your strength to the position you occupy in your business. This helps you decide on who to employ to support your business better.

Don't be a jack of all trade and mistress of none. As an individual, it helps you to build your strategic network. This is a very intentional process and you need to be very committed and deliberate about it.

4. Provide evidence: This could take the shape of success stories. Success stories are goals you've met, things you've accomplished, lessons learned, results obtained, etc. Remember, as an individual you are a brand, as a business owner, you and the business are a brand. Customers or clients could patronize your business because of you or they could leave the business for the same reason. You need to be deliberate in sharing your brand and its success.

There was this salon that I used to frequently visit and I enjoyed their services because one of the young ladies who does my manicure and pedicure is such a courteous and warm person. She would call me if she hasn't seen me for a while to know if all is well with me. On this particular day, I came into the salon wearing jeans and a T-shirt, no makeup or jewelry just looking fabulous and loving it. I greeted everyone and one of the ladies didn't respond to my greetings. I thought perhaps that she didn't hear me greet her so I repeated the greetings, this time she looked at me with such hostility and ignored me. I then ignored her and felt that she was having a bad day. I proceeded to get my nails done as usual.

The next time, I came into the salon I noticed this same woman so I didn't even bother greeting her. However this time she came to me smiling and being so nice. This got me curious, I felt that she didn't recognize me because this time around I came directly from the office and was all dressed up. As the young lady who did my manicure and pedicure was seeing me off, I asked her who the woman was and when she told me that she was the owner of the salon, I shuddered and I said I don't want to be a client of hers. This was how I negotiated for home service with the young lady.

The bottom line is this, the owner of the business lost a client because she didn't realize that she epitomizes her business. She was only nice to me when she realized my purchasing power. She provided me with evidence of how unprofessional she was and what her values are. I acted on my guiding principles and discontinued my consumption of her services.

The incident above shows how our values impact our actions or attitudes and also the relationship between values and principles.

This brings us to the final step in developing your principles. This is identifying your guiding principles.

Three Steps to Identify Your Guiding Principles

1. Guiding principles spring from your values.

2. The principles need to be consistent with the vision.

3. Guiding principles describe what experience you want people to have as a result of engaging with you or your business.

Reflect on my personal experience that I shared above and imagine that you are a business owner. What kind of experience would you want to deliver to your customers or client? As an individual when people engage with you, what experience do you want them to have?

The principles you develop are an intricate and critical aspect of your personal, career and business growth. Success is so much about the principles you live by to make your dream a reality. Your principles must be consistent with a clear vision of your dream and this guides you towards your goal.

Secret # 2: Organized

Your ability to be organized has a great impact on your success. There is rarely anyone who at one point or the other has not felt the need to be organized. The struggle to get organized is real and I know this first hand because I've gone through the episodes and from time to time, I feel the need to get more organized.

I will share with you some rules to truly organize your life and keep it organized. Then, I will show you how you can apply them across all the areas of your life that are important to you: relationships, work, finance, business, leadership etc. The result is that you will get more done while feeling less stressed. This is the point at which you really start living in abundance. I remember some years back; it was really a struggle to get all aspects of my life organized. Each time I came out, I was looking stressed, jumpy, and drained. Now, my workload has tripled but I look more relaxed. I enjoy all that I am doing. I will share a framework to help you get organized.

Rules to getting organized

Develop habits and keep routine: It's important to have set time for all your activities in a day. In this day of social media, if you wake up and the first thing you do is to grab your phone to check messages or to respond to calls, the tendency is that you will get carried away and spend more time than you have going over the phone, you will feel hurried and this kick starts your day of just jumping in and out into activities.

I will recommend that you build the habit of setting aside 20-25 minutes each morning for mediation, prayers and reflections. If you can spend more time that's great but 20-25 minutes will help set the foundation of the day. Make out time to carefully articulate your day and list your three major priorities for the day. What this does is it helps you not feel overwhelmed. I actually list a set of 3 major priorities for both my weekly and monthly priorities. This gives me room to take my time in carrying out my tasks for the day, week or month.

The main activity here is to form a habit and routine. This is the first rule in getting organized as we all have habits that have become part of our lives over years and routines that determine our actions without conscious thought.

The critical factor here is if these habits are intentional or as a result of procrastination or inertia. Good habits set us up for long-term success but building good habits isn't easy. You need to have a strong reason behind "*why*" you want to develop a certain habit. This will become your motivating factor and keep you going even when you don't feel like it.

Effective Planning: You know that there are only 24 hours in a day. Your drive should be to work smartly. This involves mapping out time for specific activities and prioritizing your daily activities.

Some of what I do are listed below:

- Map out at least 90 minutes to plan your week.

- Identify three priorities daily and be sure it's consistent with your weekly priorities.

- Overestimate how much time you require to conclude a task.

- Time block for specific activities

- Set your timer to remind you when you need to conclude certain tasks.

Organize around your uniqueness and peculiarities: When organizing, be realistic on what you can achieve. The thing is to build confidence to do more once you achieve your set targets. So schedule your tasks in achievable bits. Set targets that you can commit to in the long haul. This is called choosing the path of least resistance.

Take Daily Actions: This is where consistency is required. You need to be committed to showing up for yourself everyday once you make your commitment on the daily actions.

I got lazy over the years with my exercise and I decided to get back into shape. I scheduled twenty minutes of exercise three times a week. It was a struggle as I expected but I had committed myself to showing up three days a week and now I have progressed to 5 times a week for 40 minutes. You need to progress gradually but consistently.

Balance: There is so much you can achieve in a day. Make out time to smell the roses. Spend time with family, friends or doing what gives you so much joy. One of the greatest gifts you can give yourself is the gift of you. Your body is a machine and to perform at its optimum you need to take care of it and service it regularly. This includes good sleeping habits, eating habits, taking time away from work to rejuvenate and reflect. Stress is one of the killers of creativity. When I find myself struggling to catch up or to keep up, I know it's time for a break. Now, I have progressed to not waiting until that time but have actually started scheduling my breaks. I recognize that this is a privilege that comes with being self-employed or a boss. However, you can make this work for you. Remember no one is indispensable. I remind myself of that all the time.

One of the greatest gifts you can give your-
self is the gift of you.

Declutter: Keeping your workspace, home and other virtual and physical spaces de-cluttered is an integral aspect of staying organized. Keep your life simple. Oftentimes we are cramping so much into our lives and physical space that we begin to feel choked. Every now and again relationships and even your mind needs to be de-cluttered. You don't have to be everywhere with your friends so much so that you begin to feel pressured. Learn to use the power of the word " NO" without explanation. However, you need to be clear on the relationships and their boundaries. It's all part of decluttering. Quit being anxious and learn to do more with less.

Outsource: You can't do everything! Learn to outsource or delegate and focus on those things that you have skill sets for, things that you are passionate about and do well. Outsource or delegate the rest and do not feel guilty about it.

Measure: There is a lot of fulfillment in knowing how you've progressed. It shows what worked, what didn't and what adjustments need to be made. By measuring your progress, you are giving yourself the opportunity for more growth. You can evaluate your activities and reprioritize focusing more on those that helped you move closer towards your goals.

Be Adventurous: Finally, give yourself permission to try something new. You will be amazed at the new interests you can pick up. Consciously build adventure into your schedule and remember it is okay to let the ball drop.

Secret # 3: Wealthy

The definition of wealth is personal. What it means to be wealthy is entirely up to you. You have the ability to re-frame your reference point. It's just like success, it means different things to different people.

Henry David Thoreau was an American essayist, poet, and philosopher and he defines "wealth as the ability to truly experience life." This is the definition that I love to work with. **Wealth is beyond your financial and physical resources.** Wealth consists of every area within one's life; health, relationships, finances, time, physical possessions, human resources and more.

I will categorize wealth into four types and these are:

- Social wealth

- Time wealth

- Financial wealth

- Physical wealth

Social Wealth:

This refers to our status and is one of the most underrated types of wealth because we don't typically see our status as a form of wealth. We understand that status has value but we never make the connection that it's actually a type of wealth. Therefore we don't engage as much with our social wealth. I was having some conversations with someone a while ago and we were discussing finances and she shared how a younger brother of hers went to seek a loan from one of the local finance houses and when they got to interviewing her brother, her name came up and the interviewing officer was surprised and requested to speak with her. The loan officer said he would grant the loan to the brother if she signed the form even if her brother doesn't have collateral. She was surprised and jokingly said to me that she didn't know that her name was worth that much.

Have you done an assessment of your social wealth?

Social wealth largely comes down to how you interact within the social world. It mainly deals with what kind of character you create and how others interact with this character and perceive it.

There is one thing common to all successful and wealthy people; they have the practice of developing and maintaining relationships that form social networks willing to help each other. These networks perform best when they are diverse, so you need to identify people capable of helping your cause who you may not normally encounter or regularly interact with.

One of my priorities is to consistently grow my social capital. This facilitates my social wealth. Building the relationships that increase social capital requires time and looking at relationships as a web rather than individual connections. You need to be committed to investing your time in increasing your social capital.

Time Wealth:

This speaks to freedom and refers to the value you put on your currency of time. Time wealth is a very valuable resource and is defined as having your own time to spend how you want, where you want, and with whom you want. This is what the majority of people really want along with the other types of wealth.

Time wealth consists of understanding and mastering the fundamentals that time is finite. Developing an understanding of the importance of investing your time in building your knowledge base is critical to your growth both as an individual and a business. This specialized knowledge can be sold at a much higher rate than selling your time directly. Now rather than people buying your time, they are buying your knowledge. This affords the possibility of much more freedom and time retention. Especially as technology has created avenues for disseminating that knowledge for sale without much time being involved, i.e. selling a course online or an E -book requires no extra time once it is created and posted online.

You can increase your influence by having an understanding of how the majority of people trade time for money. Do not be limited by gender. You have been created to be all that you can imagine and even much more. You want a life of limitless possibilities? If yes, then you have to get a mastery of your time wealth.

Financial Wealth:

This is the commonly acknowledged type of wealth that is based on ownership of financial assets, such as stock, government securities, bonds and money. The acquisition of these things gives you financial freedom. It is important that you have an understanding of the fundamentals of financial wealth and how to grow your assets. You should consider options of short, mid, and long-term investments and remember, it is equally necessary to watch your spending habits. It is an unhealthy habit to spend more than what you earn. You need to enhance your financial literacy and get yourself all set up for living the life of your dreams with healthy financial habits. This means that you have to consciously allocate money to your needs and ensure that this is done judiciously. There are apps that can help you track your income, expenditure and spending habits. Picture yourself in the future where you don't have to worry about money ever again. Can you imagine the limitless possibilities this presents? Awesome yes? I tell you today that it is possible to live that life of your dream as long as you can commit to mastering financial wealth. As a P.O.W.E.R Woman you should work towards achieving all four types of wealth.

Physical Wealth: This refers to your health and body. For me, this is true wealth. Are you familiar with the saying "your health is your wealth"? The challenge is that the majority of people fail to understand this and thereby neglect to invest in their bodies and mind.

Some time back, I didn't understand the true value of taking a vacation. I would take vacations and short change myself by engaging in some type of business. I wasn't giving myself time to relax, and truly rejuvenate.

Proper nutrition, quality sleep, healthy environments, physical exercise, and health literacy are all important components of keeping your body and mind alert and effectively functioning.

How can you invest in your physical wealth more?

Now that we've discussed the various wealth categories, let's focus on the 4th secret of a power woman; which is empathy.

Secret #4: Empathetic

This is the fourth strategy that provides a life of limitless possibilities for the P.O.W.E.R Woman. Among the various lessons I learnt from Stephen's Covey book " The 7 Habits of Highly Effective People" one that stands out to me is that of empathetic listening. If you need to grow your area of influence then you need to "seek first to understand then being understood." This lesson was a major paradigm shift for me; it was a departure from my positioning of wanting people to understand my point of view. As a transformative leader, it is important that you understand the reality of the people you interact with. If you cannot wear their lenses to understand their worldview it is difficult to get them to buy into your vision. Empathy involves a deep understanding of the meaning they attribute to situations, things and an understanding of their perspective. Being empathic builds a level of trust and causes others to be more willing and open in sharing with you.

In our world, we have the habit of jumping in and trying to create solutions to challenges we do not fully understand. When I started out newly as a coach, my thinking was that it is my responsibility to create solutions to challenges. This perception changed a great deal when I engaged with the concept of " seek first to understand and then be understood." What this did for me is that it made me slower to react in a positive way, I developed the skills of allowing my clients to express themselves and their expression therein lies the solution to their challenges. I was guiding them along to dig deep, building my understanding of their uniqueness and engaging with that uniqueness for us to co-creatively come up with solutions.

Empathetic listening is one of the skills of communication that is reflected in your character. You need to be attuned to listening actively and with intent to understand the situation. This is where the paradigm shift needs to happen. You need to be committed to building the pure desire, the strength of character as well as the skill sets required for empathetic listening.

I haven't always been a very expressive person when it comes to very sensitive issues. I find more comfort writing about my feelings. Writing is very therapeutic for me. However, when I got married, it became imperative to develop effective communication skills. As I developed my verbal communication skills and learned to carefully navigate sensitive issues by trying to understand my husband's perspective before responding a lot changed positively. It doesn't mean that we don't have conflicts or that we are always on the same side of issues, but we have learnt to respect each other's perspectives even if we don't agree and try to find a middle ground in such a situation. This is partly a result of adequately understanding and using empathic communication skills.

Likewise, as you learn and build the skills to listen deeply to other people, you will discover that a shift begins to happen. The uncovering of the mind gradually takes place and you begin to inspire trust and faith in your ability to provide creative solutions. The fact is that the more you understand other people the more you will appreciate and feel respect for them. The more time you invest to deeply understand the people you love and those around you, the more dividends you get in open communication. This opens the door for you to be understood because you have built a foundation of trust, care and faith in engaging from the frame of reference of others. This is what empathy epitomizes.

Secret #5: Resilience

The ability to bounce back no matter what life throws your way defines your level of resilience. It shows how well you can deal with the difficulties of life.

Resilient people tend to maintain a more positive outlook and cope with stress more effectively. No one was born with a stockpile of resilience. This is a specialized skill set that you build as you navigate through life.

When I gave birth to my daughter and learnt that she had a fracture a few days after delivery, I was not prepared for the life changing diagnosis that we would get. When we finally got the diagnosis, it felt like a death sentence. It took a lot of effort, commitment and investment in developing my mindset for me to develop resilience. I had periods when it felt like I took one step forward, only to then take two steps backwards but I didn't let that deter me. It was all part of the resilience building process. I will share with you four strategies that helped me in building resilience and ensuring that I remained committed to enjoying my life journey. These four strategies are overcoming fear, writing, self-compassion and praying.

Strategy #1 | Overcoming Fear

When we got my daughter's diagnosis, I felt this cold feeling in the pit of my belly and it ran all over me. At first I was in denial because I didn't want to accept what the doctor was saying. It felt like a movie. I felt detached from the process after the first initial feelings. I tried to block my mind from thinking about it. This was one time in my life that I felt so scared and lonely! You know how you feel that you are the only one who understands your pain. I thank God for my husband who was so supportive through the process. I started opening my mind gradually to internalize the diagnosis. First brittle bone disease has no cure! Wow! That was huge for me and it took me time to digest that bit and get to the point of acceptance. The next question was how can I move forward? I recognized that moving forward is a process that would require my commitment and total focus if my daughter would live a near-normal life. My aha moment was my realizing that I may not have control over the disease but I have control over how I let it affect our lives. At that point, I was determined to face the future head-on. I had to let go of fear.

I recommend that you face your fears head-on but gradually. Ask yourself what is the worst that can happen? Deal with the possibilities. You can't run away from situations because you are afraid. The situation will be right there waiting for you so brace yourself. You have a choice to either to remain broken or be remolded. I chose to be remodeled into the best version of myself.

Strategy #2 | Expressive Writing

Expressive writing is simple; express how you feel with words. When I write down how I am feeling, I go to great depths to describe every bit of my feelings and reflectively write why I think I feel that way. The practice of writing helps provide clarity and move one forward by helping one gain new insights on the challenges. After writing consistently, at times up to thirty minutes or an hour. I stop and read through what I have written. I then try to find five positive things about the situation I wrote about. This becomes what I leverage on to re-write my narrative and ride out the situation.

This is a practice I do even today and I invite you to come on this writing journey with me.

Strategy #3 | Self – Compassion

When you are going through difficult or challenging times, if you are not careful, you begin to feel that you may have done something that has warranted such adversity to befall you. Then fear kicks and you wonder what exactly is wrong with you! Listen, nothing is wrong with you other than life happens. There will be good moments that make you happy and excited and there will be challenging times that make you feel sad, scared, alone and at times unwanted. It is important to recognize that everyone suffers at some point in time and that this challenging situation presents opportunities for growth. You can learn to practice self-compassion and this can be a start off to a gentle and more effective road to healing.

Self-compassion involves confronting your fears and pain with an attitude of warmth and kindness and without judgment. This involves that you are gentle and kind to yourself, you are very deliberate with what you feel and say, you remember that this is normal and that you are not alone. You also need self-acceptance and compassion toward yourself about a specific struggle/ pain without feeling ashamed or guilty. Finally, look for the silver lining in the situation and make a commitment to yourself to consider constructive ways to improve in the future.

Strategy #4 | Praying

I deeply believe in the power of prayer and my faith in God the creator of the universe is what has brought me this far. I remember immersing myself in prayers and desperately searching for answers to my daughter's situation in the scriptures. I got more than I bargained for. I developed a very personal relationship with God. I became more spiritual rather than more religious, I sought to understand situations and people better without making any judgments. I have confessed several times that initially, I was so upset with God at the beginning of my fourteen years journey of nurturing my daughter. I look back now and I am not filled with regret at my actions for those feelings and actions because it is what drew me into a more personal relationship with God.

I won't dwell too much on prayers because the whole of this book speaks to the power of prayers in building your resilience. I encourage you to discover God for yourself. Allow Him to introduce Himself to you like He did to me and I promise you that your life will change for the best.

The five secrets that I have shared with you in this chapter if practiced mindfully will astronomically increase your circle of influence and open up opportunities of living a life of limitless possibilities. Do not be afraid of failures but be terrified of living a life of regrets. Give yourself permission to play full out. Barriers, challenges, pain and failures should motivate you to seek for alternative solutions.

You can be the **BEST VERSION** of yourself if only you are willing to play full out and ready to come out of your shell. Remember the world awaits for you to come forth and shine your light so brightly that it illuminates the pathway of those around you. This is your moment; the time can never be perfect.

P.O.W.E.R WOMAN! The world is your stage. Rule your world.

5

Transforming Your Mindset to Achieve Your Goals

*"Your mindset is one of the most valuable
assets that you have and you need to guard
it jealously. "*

Y ou can channel the power and energy of your mind towards achieving your goals and living your dream life if you can transform your mindset and find a more empowering meaning in life. Your thoughts are created in the framework of your mind, your thoughts shape your reality and how you experience life thereby making your mindset one of the most powerful tools you can ever imagine. The way you perceive a situation as challenging or empowering, frustrating or a learning opportunity all depends on your mindset. This is why you need to pay attention to developing your mindset and harnessing its full potential. If you are able to harness the full potential of your mindset then you are ready to experience an unforgettable limitless life. When it comes to transforming your mind, like anything else, it takes time and consistent efforts to build your capacity.

To transform your life, you need to change how you think and to do this you need to learn how to transform your mindset. Broadly there are two types of mindset, the growth mindset and the fixed mindset. Growth-mindset people take on challenges and are open to learning from failures. They understand that failures are the building block of a successful life. This is from the understanding that talent can be cultivated through efforts. Whereas fixed-mindset people are not prone to learning new ways of being, they get discouraged when something requires significant effort and failure is like a death sentence to them.

What makes growth-mindset more likely to be successful? Growth-mindset people define success by stretching to learn something new. They understand that success is about doing your best, constantly improving, learning and defining your success frame of reference. One of the key attributes of a growth mindset is the power to avoid labels. It is important to know that labels can create limiting thoughts and stop people from taking steps to achieve their goals. Labels could either be positive or negative.

Some examples of labels are "not smart enough", "intelligent", "high-flyer", etc. Positive labels can stop people taking risks because they fear failure and they want to be consistent with their positive label. I was having a conversation with a friend and we were discussing our children and the expectations that they have of us. My friend mentioned an incident that happened once during the sports day at her children's school. There was a call for parents to have a running competition. Her children were urging her to join the race, she said that looking at the excitement on their faces a fleeting thought crossed her mind; what if she doesn't win this race, she would have ended up crushing the excitement for her children and with that thought she refused to join the race. One thing struck me, she was fixated on the fact that her children wanted her to win the race but what if for the children it was simply the pleasure of having their mum participate and cheering her on. That was an opportunity to reverse the role and give her children the opportunity of encouraging her. She was more fixated on not disrupting the positive perception her children had of her running abilities. Can you imagine the excitement those kids would have had? It is beyond " winning " or " losing". When we get fixated on labels we miss opportunities that situations present for us to stretch ourselves. Failures are painful for everybody, but the truth is that failure does not define you. It is a problem to be faced, to be dealt with and to learn from. It is an opportunity to learn. I see failure as a process of learning from your mistakes. If you are invested in learning, you need to evaluate your current abilities, know the gaps and be open and willing to be vulnerable in order to learn effectively. This also implies that you are open to constructive criticism. Learning is about the process, about what has been accomplished through practice, study, persistence, choices and good strategy. The process is as important as the end result.

Growth mindset people are willing to be vulnerable to experience challenging situations. In a growth-mindset challenges are motivating, informative and an opportunity to develop. One question that will help you in knowing if you need to work on your mindset is the answer to this question: Are you regularly accomplishing your goals and living your dreams? If you answered "yes," by now you can identify why this is so and if you said "no," I would share some of the life changing strategies that worked for me.

I strongly encourage you to pick at least three from the list below and commit to applying it on a daily basis. Remember to be clear about how you will practice it and to track your progress so that you can monitor your progress and consistency!

Strategy # 1 | Mindfulness

Accept that your thinking needs adjusting, remember if your thinking changes then your life becomes transformed. We've all had goals and dreams that didn't unfold the way we hoped or expected. When this happens repeatedly, we start to wonder what we need to change. But rarely do we look inside at our own thinking as the place to start making changes. Your change should be from the inside out. That is when sustainable transformation begins to happen.

It is equally critical to pay attention and notice your thoughts as well as the words that you use to describe a situation, yourself or whatever might be happening around you. The words you use can be the trigger for how your mind will interpret its meaning and subsequently how you feel about it. For instance, the first two years of my daughter's life whenever she had one of her frequent fractures, I would lament, cry, and I felt so miserable and helpless. By the time I started engaging with the power of transforming my mindset, when her fractures happen, I saw it as an opportunity to show her how much she is loved and to build her resilience. Today despite her physical limitations, she is one of the happiest children that I have come across. So the first step in transforming your mindset is to simply acknowledge that you're going to work on your mindset and be more intentional of your thoughts and words. This will help you to have more empowering thoughts, channel your thoughts towards something more inspiring and encouraging, and to be able to find solutions or understand a situation differently.

Strategy # 2 | Remain Positive

Let's be honest, there are some days that no matter how much you try it's very challenging to channel your thoughts to a more empowering place. This can be for various reasons, perhaps too much stress at work or a major disagreement with your spouse. In those instances, I find that I need to push myself to the extra level to remain positive. I do everything that I can to cut out the negative noise or flood it out of my head. One of the strategies that work for me is listening to uplifting gospel music that reminds me of God's faithfulness and plan for my life. I got my daughter into joining me in this practice and we would sing and pray together. Sometimes we break into tears. I can tell you that remaining positive is a choice that I have chosen even when I don't seem to understand situations, I take consolation in the fact that everything will work out for my good. This is a very simple but empowering choice. The fact is that I am redirecting my mind towards something more inspiring and empowering than pondering on the thoughts and emotions that I'm feeling. This gives me the boost to make a move even when I feel weighed down.

I strongly encourage you to find out what works for you. Whatever tools work for you, do it until you feel better and have more energy and focus to be able to assess and redirect your mindset.

Strategy # 3 | Identify and Overcome Your Fears

Mindsets are formed through prior experiences and emotional milestones. These experiences could have created some self-doubt, limiting beliefs, and any other negative thoughts that get in the way of your fulfillment. Sometimes we hear that little but persistent voice that reminds us of all our failures and tells us that we are not good enough. We all know that voice. It makes you hesitate before approaching someone you'd like to meet. It makes you think twice before starting a business or considering a career change.

It's hard to remain positive when that little voice keeps blabbing and reminding you all of the negative things you will rather forget. The way to overcome that voice is to identify your fears and your limiting thoughts because you can't change what you haven't acknowledged. Once they've been identified you need a way to stop them from holding you back. One of the best strategies that I know for this is something I call "worse case scenario".

During the early years of my daughter's life, when I had all kinds of fears because of her condition, I identified the fears and knew that if I was to move forward I had to find a way of overcoming my fears. For each of my fears I would ask myself what is the worst-case scenario? I would then ask myself if I was comfortable living a life of regrets not knowing for certain that the worst case scenario would even be the end result. This was a game changer for me. Here's an even deeper example, when I think that I'm not good enough, instead of allowing it to limit me, it becomes my energizer. I see the worst case scenario of not knowing and then switch it by learning, obtaining more information on the subject matter. Now the worse case scenario isn't even an option and I've opened myself up to the possibility of learning through failing. In turn, I have broadened my experience. I had a consultancy a little over ten years ago to run a specialized training for a client. The curriculum for the training went so well but I ran into troubled waters with the logistics. It was so huge that I lost all my funds and even went into debt, that I never imagined that I could come out of it. While I was trying to wade out of the situation, I was scared to take on further consultancies because I was scared of failing. I had lost confidence in my abilities. However, at the same time I needed to have more jobs so that I could work out a payment plan. I was scared of even confronting the magnitude of the mess that I was in. It took me several efforts to sit and reflect on the situation and to acknowledge the depth of my situation. I was able to identify what I should have done better; this became a building block to the success I enjoy today. I can handle consultancies and projects running into multi -million dollars. Aside that, I have built my skill sets in other relevant areas that identified as the gap in the major loss that I experienced.

It is not a quick fix but you need to be committed to the journey of transformation. Often, just taking one positive step in the right direction is enough to shut those fears and build your confidence No one was born with a reservoir of confidence, you build it gradually by small wins and then you feel embolden to expand your risk taking and you get to the level where you can spring back no matter what.

Strategy # 4 | Mentorship and Coaching

We are all on different levels and paths on our personal growth journey. There are moments that you are able to uplift someone else, but there are moments where you need a bit of a helping hand. You've got to know that it is perfectly okay. It doesn't mean that anything is wrong with you, it simply acknowledges that you are human.

For instance, where you are struggling to change your mindset and redirect your thoughts, I find that talking to someone who is able to have a more positive mindset can help you talk through the emotions you are feeling, and guide you to a more empowering and positive mindset. This is where having a mentor or a coach is very helpful. I have two coaches, one for my personal growth and another for business development and finances. When I hit a brick wall, or if I feel that I need support or encouragement, I draw from their wealth of experience.

Sometimes, you just need to talk through whatever you are feeling to be able to let it go, gain clarity and to develop a more empowering mindset. With practice, this becomes easier with time and you will be able to transform your mindset.

Strategy # 5 | Understand your "why"

Changing your mindsets takes work because formed habits aren't easy to break. Understanding your "why" is about your purpose, it gives you deeper insight into yourself and a larger perspective on what makes you unique. It is about connecting with what you are passionate about. Your " why" means understanding why you do the things you do! It's your reason for being passionate and motivated. Your " WHY" is as unique as your fingerprint. It drives you to be focused and when you are so committed to it, your impact and influence grow.

To understand your " why" you need to dig deep to find out what your priorities are and which one means so much to you. I do what I do because I love to put smiles on the faces of people, inspire people to discover themselves and be the best version of themselves. This is my why. I am constantly looking for ways to inspire people to greatness. It gives me so much satisfaction. I want you to reflect on your " why" if you don't know what it is , it is difficult for you to remain motivated enough to achieve your set goals. Once you identify what your "why" is, write it down. Why does it really matter to you and then mediate on that. You will be surprised at what this uncovers. This is an important part of building your motivation and staying motivated. Your " why" becomes your driving force. Often I get questions like, " how do you do all that you do? How do you find the time and energy? My response is that I am living out my purpose and this is the life of my dreams. I sleep, wake up and act, focused on my passion. I am completely invested in it. It hasn't always been this way. I was at some point in my life drifting and seeking for answers and once I got it there was no stopping me. I learned how to be consistent in the pursuit of my "why".

Strategy #6 | Consistency

High achievers understand the importance of starting small and finishing big. Be willing to get started, it is one of the best ways to change your mindsets and realize your dreams. Set micro and achievable goals. This builds your confidence to keep pushing. Starting small enables you to take daily consistent actions. Decide that your micro goal is the minimum, and that you can achieve it. A lot of the time, you'll do more and will feel great because you're overachieving. Some days you may do the minimum, and you'll still feel great because you've met your goal. Most importantly, you are taking daily consistent actions. Over time, consistently hitting your micro goals will form new mindset habits, and that's real progress toward transforming your thinking so you can reach your biggest dreams.

Strategy # 7 | Get Comfortable with Failure

The strategies for transforming your mindset that I've outlined so far will help you move forward with confidence toward achieving more of your goals and living a limitless life of possibilities. However, it's critical to understand that it will be hard work and there will be building blocks (failures) along the way. Most times when people hit a brick wall, they give up, make an excuse or are scared to try again. Successful people realize that the only thing that will keep them from their goals is to stop trying, so they never stop trying! No matter how long it takes, they keep their focus. They know that it is normal to encounter obstacles and even fail several times along the way.

However, they are prepared for the barriers and are committed to breaking the barriers no matter what. They know it's coming, and it doesn't scare them or make them give up. **When failure happens, they reflect, seek feedback, learn valuable lessons and make adjustments that will keep them moving forward.**

You too can do this by giving yourself permission to fail (build blocks of success). It will take the pressure off getting a perfect end result.

Transforming your mindset doesn't happen by accident, it can't be a coincidence, it is an intentional choice, and these 7 strategies outlined above should help get you on the right track.

6

Stay Focused Power Woman

Staying Focused is one of the principles of success. All extraordinary achievements require a clear focus and to achieve your goals, you need to learn techniques to stay focused and practice them with effort and dedication. Staying focused on your goals is not an easy task as there are several distractions that are competing for your time. In the beginning, when planning your goals there is a high level of energy and you are motivated. But over time when the pressures of life come knocking, we get caught up, stuck, overloaded, frustrated, distracted, and we simply just go off track. Our motivation takes a dip and the struggle to stay focused begins.

It is easy to get inundated by emergencies and crises that feel almost unavoidable, so losing that all-important focus feels largely, well, unimportant. Yet, in the back of our minds, we know that these are surmountable excuses and if we are to live the life of our dream we need to keep our eyes on the ball and stay focused on our goals.

I have gotten frustrated with my progress towards my goals in the past, so I understand what it feels like. It is not an easy process to keep yourself from distractions or from going off track but then nothing good comes easy. Staying focused on your goals requires mastering some techniques to help you keep your eyes on the ball. This requires developing an effective plan to stay focused, and to help you anticipate those time-wasters and things that tend to take you off your goals.

There are some very effective methods that you can employ to help you keep your focus on your goals. I will encourage you to pick two or three that resonates with you, make a plan and remain committed to stick to that plan.

Strategy #1 | Create a Mission Statement

Your personal mission statement is the first step in articulating what your end results will look like. It describes what you want to be, your achievements and contributions. The mission statement should help direct your time and energy towards the things that matter most to you and help you stay focused on those all-important goals. It articulates what you value, what you believe in and what you want to accomplish. It details your uniqueness, personal value proposition and how you do things differently than others. When you get distracted or lose your focus, re-read your mission statement and re-envision why you're doing what you're doing on a daily basis.

I will strongly recommend that you create a detailed mission statement in 4 or 5 sentences and hang it somewhere you can see it every single day.

Strategy #2 | Write out your goals

Write out your goals. Your goals should embody your values and what you are set out to accomplish, and be sure that it is consistent with your mission statement. Brainstorm and write down everything you want to achieve. Look at your lists and group items that are similar or that can be combined into one larger goal. Look at your simplified goals and circle the ones you feel are your highest priority. Looking at your priorities, identify one to two major goals that will make the biggest impact on your life. Always approach the most important goals first. If you want to stay focused on your goals, then you need to ensure you're tackling them in the right way. If you're serious about your goals, then you have to actively set and detail them out. Ensure that your goals are SMART- specific, measurable, achievable, realistic and time bound.

Specific: Is your goal(s) something that could be easily identified when you've reached it? If not, how could you make it more specific?

Measurable: Would you be able to tell you've reached it? Is there a clear criteria? If not, how could you make it more measurable?

Achievable: Is your goal(s) achievable? Is it something that you've considered and understand that it is, in fact, possible and able to be accomplished? If not, how could you adjust your goal and/or timeframe expectations to make it achievable?

Realistic: Is your goal(s) realistic? Is it something you are:

a) Physically and mentally capable of doing

b) Prepared for, and

c) Able to commit to?

If not, is there another way to reach your goal or something you can do to put this one within reach?

Time Bound: Does your goal(s) have a time frame? Have you set a date or duration? Do you have timelines for the next step? If not, is there anything else you need to do in order to be able to put your goal on a timeline and begin taking action?

Strategy #3 | Develop milestones towards your goals

Sometimes, it's hard to stay focused on our goals because they seem so far off. It is far easier if you can create a set of milestones towards your goals. Develop a set of milestones that will help you move towards your goals without losing your focus. To create your milestones, just break down your goals into equal parts. Carefully construct a set of milestones that will help you move forward towards achieving your goals.

Strategy #4 | Develop and follow a plan

To stay focused on our goals, we need a plan. A plan is what helps move us from where we are to where we want to go. Having an effective plan helps you to take action towards achieving your goals on a daily basis.

You should create a mid term and long-term plan to help you reach your goals, but it should have some flexibility to accommodate changes along the way. What shouldn't change are your goals. You can reach your goals as long as you can follow a plan. If you see the plan isn't working, all you have to do is slightly change your direction. It doesn't take much. But it does take time and consistency.

Strategy #5 | Effective Time Management

It's virtually impossible to stay focused on your goals if you can't manage your time. It is important that you chose a time management system that works and is adaptable to your uniqueness. One of the best ones out there is the quadrant time management system. It splits your daily activities up into four separate quadrants based on two factors: 1) urgency, and 2) importance.

The plan is to stay away from time-wasting activities, which are not urgent and not important (quadrant 4). It's easy to lose focus on your goals when you're engaged in this quadrant for much of the day, which includes things like excessively using social media, over-socializing with friends etc.

To stay focused on your goal you need to spend as much of your day in the not-urgent-but-important quadrant (quadrant 2), which includes your long-term goals. Our long-term goals are never urgent in the here-and-now, but they are important to our lives.

Strategy #6 | Measuring Progress

One crucial way you can stay focused on your goals is to track and analyze your progress. Set a measurable goal, track it, and be honest with the result. It's the only way you'll know whether you're growing—or not. In fact, how else would you know just how far you've come towards achieving your goals or just how much there's left to go?

Measuring and tracking your progress is the route to goal success and staying focused on your goals over time. There are different apps on your smartphone to help you in daily tracking or you can simply use a spreadsheet on your laptop to plot your results on a daily basis. The more data you have, the more you can analyze and determine just which of your efforts are paying off and which ones needed to be readjusted or discarded.

Strategy #7 | Avoid Procrastination

The last, but certainly not least, method for staying focused on your goals is to avoid procrastination. I am also guilty of procrastination, and truth be told we sometimes have doses of procrastination periodically. It is not so simple to stay focused sometimes you just feel like postponing that action until a later time, or you find some excuses for not getting the task done. I remember how much effort it took me to get started on my daily exercises. I was always coming up with one excuse or the other to justify my procrastination. To get doing and me up and focused on achieving my goals I had to put some strategy in place. One simple way to do this is to use the 15-minutes rule. Simply grab your smartphone or a timer and set it to 15 minutes. The idea behind the 15 minutes is that we can all do something for 15 minutes. I started encouraging myself to commit to doing my exercise for only 15 minutes three times a week. What happens is that most times I go on to 30 minutes and now I commit to more than 15 minutes per exercise time. I will encourage you to try this strategy. Commit to doing whatever it is that you've been putting off for 15 minutes, no more. Once the 15 minutes is up, you can choose to stop or if you have become sucked into the process, keep going and, even if you stop, you at least break the seal. You stopped procrastinating, even if it was only for a short while. Since habits take time to form or break, this is an important step in the art of habit formation. So, the 15 minute-rule is a perfect pattern disruption technique.

You need to remain committed to staying focused because at the end of the day it's up to you to stay focused on your goals, and not someone else. The only person you would be cheating by not putting in the effort every single day to achieve your goals, is yourself. Don't be afraid of failure. Always be too focused to give up! And make time to play. It's important to smell the roses as you travel on your path. That's the spirit of a Power Woman.

7

No Matter What

*"What's the essence of my voice if I can't use
it to impact on lives? What's the joy of living
if I can't connect to inspire and be inspired
by the journey of others?"*

If you say that you are going to do something no matter what, you are emphasizing that you are definitely going to do it, even if there are obstacles or difficulties. This is the transformed mindset that you need to develop and push forward with. It is imperative that you acknowledge that the path to growing your circle of influence and becoming a power woman. It is not an easy one and you need to commit to giving all that it takes to achieve your dreams and goals. The difference that a power woman brings to the table is her unflinching resolution to keep pushing until she achieves her goals. These days there are a number of distractions, (some are legitimate) which can make you give excuses or simply give up when you hit a brick wall. I encourage you to be completely sold out on your dreams. Take the stance that no matter what may come up, "I will not let go of my dreams." Believe that you are enough to achieve your dream. You do not need the validation of anyone to keep your focus. Know this, many people who condemn and judge you for actions you take, secretly wish they could have the same boldness as you. Keep your focus on " You ". The vision is yours' and do not expect that people will understand your vision. The fear of not being enough, not having the prerequisite skills to carry out a task, waiting for affirmations or validations form certain persons that you hold in high esteem and the list keeps getting long. This is just a distraction, stay focused.

There was a time in my life that I was afraid to take certain actions to move myself forward because I was waiting for certain persons to play catch up or because I was feeling guilty at leaving other people behind. I have grown to realize that we all have different callings and sometimes even when we are on the same journey our purposes are different. So stepping away from the crowd and being you is not a crime and needs no validation but give yourself full permission to play full out. The process of the journey is just as important as the destination. It is in the process you build certain habits that determine how long you can have the " no matter what " attitude. It is important to pay attention to details so that you don't get burnt out or you do not lose your way on your journey. Sometimes we know in parts and as we grow in our purpose, a number of insights are gained and this changes the course of journey, we simply learn to take a different route.

Being scared of being visible is a real thing. I know because I once was scared of being visible. I would always want to hide in the background and operate from there. Along the way I made a ton of mistakes and lost faith. It took the birth and nurturing process of my amazing daughter for me to discover me and then I started living on my own terms.

I developed a breakthrough mindset that enabled me to make actionable plans and take consistent efforts for my personal and business breakthroughs. I started out as a young woman seeking to discover her voice. One thing I didn't take into consideration when I started my journey of discovery was the influence I would have as I serve people.

This was the biggest transformation that I faced growing from a woman seeking clarity to one exuding so much confidence and wearing lots of caps, having a voice that is heard and the ability to influence people's choices. As a breakthrough coach and personal growth influencer, I've had the privilege of holding the hands of many women as they de- clutter and untangle themselves from limiting beliefs and barriers. I get to help women on a daily basis to move beyond their challenge, feel more confident and live life on their terms.

As a transformative leader, I inspire women to achieve remarkable results by teaching them how to identify needed change and to create a vision to guide the change. I am driven to work with passionate women who are willing to give themselves the permission to play full out. And when I get comments, mails, DMs from followers or clients telling me I've changed their lives that for me is the real WIN.

It Is Okay to Drop the Ball

I've had my fair share of looking back in regret at some aspects of my life and wishing that I could change some of the decisions that I made or undo some actions . The truth is there is no guarantee that I would have a different outcome. Living a life of regret is one way the accuser of the brethren torments us and blocks us from living a life of Joy . You can't keep looking back in regret. There are no guarantees in life. All that is assured is the present. The future remains an uncharted course that we have to navigate. Life constantly evolves and you have no control over that. However, you have control over your decisions and actions so remain focused and lean not upon your own understanding.

At times a shift needs to occur for you to unleash the power inside. This may entail moving out of your comfort zone and wearing the cloak of resilience. You may be tempted to believe that God has abandoned you, or that you are on the wrong path. Do not give up; keep holding on for sometimes you need to step out to step into something greater. You need to understand that it is okay to drop the ball. That is why you are human.

You may have engaged in a number of business ventures and they've all crumpled. Perhaps you took a loan and it still didn't come through. You may have lost everything? Your debtors are closing in and you are so scared to make another move.

You are not alone!

I've gone through such situations and I can relate with your fears. When the ball drops, it may be a sign that you are exhausted and need to take a rest or that you need to reflect and re-strategize. It could be that a more creative approach is needed. Be willing to learn the lessons from each process and do not be afraid of the ball dropping because it will drop countless times and you need to build your resilience in picking up the ball and getting back in the game.

Do Not Give Up

There was a time in my life when I wasn't as confident as I am right now. I wasn't clear on what I really wanted. After I got married, I worked in my husband's company for some years, then the economy took a turn for the worse and between the high cost of production and incredibly dishonest staff we had to close the company after painfully struggling. We imported materials for producing weavons and wigs, tried our hands on the new production line for a while and we couldn't break even. At this time I was seriously feeling so frustrated because we had lost a lot in the whole process but giving up wasn't on the table. It seemed that the more failures I encountered the more I became more determined to break the cycle. My husband and I decided to invest in ovulation kits, we got affiliated to a production company in Canada and we marketed in Nigeria. This took off well until our distributor began sourcing a cheaper, less efficient product. This impacted our sales and with time it wasn't profitable selling our brand anymore. I then went into selling women clothing. I would travel to the UK to buy clothes and accessories. I would end up selling all my goods but few customers paid and it was so much pain trying to collect payments and most importantly I wasn't passionate about the process. I tried network marketing and I was convinced that it's not for me. This whole process helped shape my understanding of who I am and what drives me.

Along the way I took an interest in raising awareness on cervical cancer and so I started an awareness campaign on Cervical Cancer and I discovered that I love imparting knowledge and women having new understanding of their agency inspired me. This kick-started my journey in the development space. The more I got involved the more I was loving the space and evolving. I had discovered my purpose through a series of failures. If I had given up, I may not be where I am today. I look back at how far I've come and how much I've been able to impact on my world and I am filled with a sense of deep gratitude. I've stepped into my light and I am not dimming it. It's been over twenty years of progressively hard work, committed investments in training, coaching and capacity building retreats. I have a mantra "too focused to give up." This has made me to be focused and very intentional.

I have a strong belief that every obstacle must be surmounted or dismantled. I don't wait until the situation is perfect or the environment is ready. I make an attempt and strive to soar above limitations. I've had failures that made me cringe or want to give up but I made a commitment to myself that no matter what, I'll keep pushing on because I have a purpose to fulfill. Each "Failure" marked the beginning of my success. I look back in deep gratitude to God who blessed my efforts. It's been a consistent growth path, a journey I wouldn't trade for another.

Do I have my out and down moments? Of course I do. For I am human but I've learnt to pick myself up, dust off and move on for I am too focused to give up. I'm grateful that I don't look anything like what I've been through.

Stop Putting it Off

I know that there have been challenges too numerous to recount but you have the opportunity of making empowering choices. There are actions that you need to get started on. It starts from your mind. Make the shift. You can't keep putting off your purpose. It's okay if you fall, it's okay to decide to crawl instead of walking but you need to get started. One baby step at a time will push you off in the right directions.

Power Woman, have confidence in your skills and capacity and never apologize for being you. Always remember to celebrate you and refuse to be defined by people. Set your standards and definition of living and show others how to value and treat you. Be ready to serve for in service you find fulfillment. Seek quality friendships and undiluted loyalty and remember to celebrate sisters who have made an impact in your life.

Finally, make God the centerpiece of your life and watch Him water and grow YOU beyond your wildest imagination.

8

It's Time to Take That Leap

"Do what you can, with what you have, where you are."

- Theodore Roosevelt

You can't keep procrastinating on taking the necessary actions for you to move forward. There are points in your life when you are called to take a leap of faith. You want to do something that is positive for your life, but you're afraid that it may not work out the way you want. You may be worried that you don't know exactly how to do it and you don't want to make a mistake.

They are times in our lives when our inner voice is asking us to make change happen, and if we do, then our lives can elevate to the next level. But fear often rears up so intensely that it threatens to kill that possibility!

I remember this only too well. In 2007, at that point in my life, I had been nurturing my daughter who was having frequent fractures and I couldn't trust anyone else to care for her, of course what this entailed was that I was always by her side. My life came to a halt. I knew I wanted to do something new and interesting, but I was scared of taking a step forward for then I didn't particularly like being outside my comfort zone, which was by my daughter's side. Well, the truth is, I preferred doing what I was already good at, which is caring and nurturing my daughter and I wasn't ready to confront the unknown.

When it comes to doing something new in your life, you prepare as much as possible but there is only so much preparation you can do. There comes a point when you've prepared, and then you realize that you are scared. You are confronted with some questions that you will never get answers to for example, "What is going to happen?" and "Will this work out?" This makes you develop cold feet to taking the leap of faith. This is where trust comes into play. You need to trust that you are enough to take that leap. This is not blind faith. It's an innate, deep knowing and a passion that draws you forward. It demands that you invest in faith and trust yourself to surmount all obstacles.

What Do You See?

You came into your new season with something in your hands. In Exodus 4:2 (NIV) God asked Moses "What is in your hands?" Moses felt he had nothing but a rod! He was scared to go on the mission of liberating the Israelites because he saw himself as a mere shepherd. He didn't believe that he could command the Israelites' attention not to talk of the King of Egypt. Moses's ordinary rod was turned into a snake before the King!

How do you see yourself? Have you allowed other people's definition of you or the circumstances you find yourself in to limit your expectations or to dim your light? I confidently tell you that it doesn't matter the size or quantity of what is in your hands. You can take inspired actions to grow or expand that which you have in your hands once you take the leap of faith. It however depends on what you see. What you see influences the actions and decisions you make. Do you see a mountain or a ladder? Do you see challenges or an opportunity to learn to depend on God? Do you see betrayal or a choice to let go of a toxic relationship? Do you see singleness or the privilege of discovering and growing yourself? Do you see scarcity or abundance?

You may need to get a new pair of lenses to see the opportunities and unlimited possibilities around you. When we look around at all the things we wish we could impact—both in our own life and the world around us—it's easy to feel overwhelmed. But you've had the rod in your hands the entire time; it's what you do with it that makes the difference.

You see, one of the most surprising secrets about stepping into your true calling is that you'll likely find yourself making a real impact on the world around you in a unique way that only you can fulfill.

This will look different for everyone, and it might not look like you expect it to. But when you follow this path, it will happen. And you will find joy on this path, for nothing fulfills us more authentically and deeply than living in alignment with our purpose. It's time to bring everything you have to the table right now. To wake up and contribute to the reality you want to create so as to live and enjoy your true calling.

We make the difference when we own our voice and live purposefully then we can impact on others positively. Empowered women transform societies.

Look At Me Now

One of the lessons that I have learnt on my personal growth journey is that I need to have faith in myself. Power Woman, it's time to remember who you really are! You are powerful and there is no failing when you leap. Someone who leaps is always a winner. It's time to take that leap of faith; knowing that He who calls you is faithful and will never let you fall. In your weakness, God's strength is made abundant. Though people may have given up on you and questioned your very existence, remember the potter molds the clay for a purpose.

It's time to rise up for you, perfect just as you are, beautifully and wonderfully made in the image of the Most High. Welcome to a new beginning and new season. You are ready to be a power woman. And I am right here with you!

PROFILE OF DR. JOY ADA ONYESOH

Dr. Joy Ada Onyesoh is the International President of the Women's International League for Peace and Freedom (WILPF), Country Director of Women's International League for Peace and Freedom (WILPF) Nigeria and President and Founder of Joy Onyesoh Foundation (JOF).

Dr.Joy Onyesoh has been an active member of WILPF since 2007, in 2011, she became the convener of the WILPF Africa working group and in 2014, and she became the International Vice President and the African liaison of WILPF. On the 22nd of August 2018, during the historic 32nd Triennial International Congress of WILPF, Dr. Joy Ada Onyesoh was elected as the International President. This is historic as she is the youngest, first black and African to hold the office of the International President of the 104 years organization and the oldest international women's peace organization in the world.

Dr. Joy Onyesoh is an alumnus of the prestigious Golda Meir MASHAV Carmel International Training Centre Israel and the Women's Human Rights Institute, University of Toronto Canada. She has also earned several certificates in Transformative leadership, women and peace building and Women Empowerment amongst others. She is a public speaker and International Best Selling Author. Joy is the convener of SHE SPEAKS and Broken But Remoulded . She is a Breakthrough and Transformative leadership coach for passion driven women who have a need to discover their purpose and thrive as a result of gaining clarity on ways of creating unlimited abundance.

Her mission is to serve passionate women who are willing to unlock their potentials for growth, build confidence in the face of uncertainty and are desirous to experience a life of unlimited abundance . Joy is a passionate, self motivated individual with a drive to succeed, having excellent organizational and interpersonal skills. She is a woman of many parts, highly efficient, methodical and with a proactive approach to performance. Her slogan is " Too Focused to Give Up", and this drives her passion in making a difference in the lives of others. Joy's purpose is to inspire greatness in others and to help people find their life's purpose and live an impactful life. She creates opportunities for women and girls to find and own their voice. A Rotarian and a Paul Harris Fellow of Rotary International, Joy has a large heart for service towards humanity.

Dr. Joy Onyesoh has also received several organizational and International awards for her role in promoting women empowerment and the most recent is the 2019 Female Civility Award for her commitment to women's empowerment globally.

For speaking engagements or interviews contact Dr. Joy Onyesoh at joyonyesoh@joyonyesoh.com